THE POWER BOOSTERS

Minerals like zinc, chromium and copper are vital to human nutrition—but by their very nature are hard to assimilate in the body. They need "transport service" from other substances, known as chelators, and new research is showing that one of the most effective chelating agents is picolinic acid, a natural constituent of living cells. This Good Health Guide, prepared by one of the pioneers of that research, shows how picolinates—mineral-picolinic acid compounds—are multiplying the nutrient effectiveness of essential minerals and preventing health-threatening deficiencies.

ABOUT THE AUTHOR

Gary W. Evans, Ph.D. is Professor of Chemistry at Bemidji State University in Minnesota, where he performed much of the research described in this Good Health Guide. He is the author of many professional articles and papers and has contributed to several books.

THE PICOLINATES

HOW THEY HELP BUILD MUSCLE WITHOUT STEROIDS—AND THEIR OTHER HEALTH BENEFITS

by Gary W. Evans, Ph.D.

Keats Publishing, Inc. New Canaan, Connecticut

The Picolinates is not intended as medical advice. Its intention is solely informational and educational. Please consult a medical or health professional should the need for one be indicated.

THE PICOLINATES

ISBN: 0-87983-511-7

Printed in the United States of America

Good Health Guides are published by
Keats Publishing, Inc.
27 Pine Street (Box 876)
New Canaan, Connecticut 06840

Contents

INTRODUCTION

Aware of the deteriorating quality of our diet, I began, about 20 years ago, searching for the most efficient ways to supplement daily diets with essential metals. The United States Department of Agriculture supported and funded much of that research. My work, in conjunction with my associates, culminated in the discovery of a metal chelator that can and should be used by the general public. That chelator is picolinic acid, which easily combines with mineral elements to make what are called metal picolinates.

The metal picolinate of zinc—zinc picolinate—lowers the daily dietary needs for zinc by at least half. The metal picolinate of chromium makes the job of the hormone insulin much easier. Chromium picolinate given to diabetics causes the glucose level in the blood to decrease. When people with high blood levels of cholesterol take chromium picolinate orally, the blood cholesterol goes down. Also, chromium picolinate speeds up the development of muscles in athletes.

Metal picolinates are extremely effective because, unlike chelators used in medicine and sold in health food stores, *picolinic acid is produced by the body for improving the passage of metal ions into the cells.* Fortunately, metal picolinates are safe as well as easy and relatively inexpensive to produce, and can be used by the general public to prevent metal deficiencies in the body.

Minerals such as zinc, chromium, iron and copper are needed inside the body so that the machinery of the cells always works efficiently and at a maximum capacity. A problem, however, is that these elements cannot be made by the body and are not even stored very efficiently in the body. Therefore, mineral elements must be constantly delivered to the cells from an outside source—the food we eat.

The wall around the castle. However, in order for the minerals to pass from our food to the cells where they are needed, they must pass through several barriers. These barriers are made up of the chemicals that surround the cells to form a protective wall called the membrane. These walls are not easily penetrated and often completely reject any element or chemical compound that does not have the correct makeup. In other words, the cell membranes are like the walls around a medieval castle. Without proper documentation, visitors are turned away. In the case of the mineral elements, they often stand the chance of being turned away because they carry with them an electrical charge that cannot be carried inside the cell. Thus, for the mineral elements to enter the cells, they must first surrender their charge. This can be done if the mineral element travels with a chemical companion that itself uses the chemical charge and makes it possible for the element to enter the cell. These chemical traveling companions are called chelators.

Chelation: A means to penetrate the wall and enter the castle. To understand why picolinic acid is the chelator of choice in nature, we should first review what is meant by chelation and why it is necessary. The word "chelate" comes from a Greek word meaning "claw." Chelators are chemicals that hold other chemicals as in a claw. For metal chelators, the other chemical is a metal. More accurately, the other chemical is a metal ion, because metals are only found in the body in a charged form that chemists call ions. All the elements that make up our universe contain small positive particles called protons, which are surrounded by rings of negative particles called electrons.

When the number of protons and electrons is equal, there is no charge and these elements are called atoms. However, in many elements, particularly metals, one or two or sometimes three electrons are found circling around the outer perimeter of the element. Because these electrons are on the perimeter, they are not held very tightly and they escape. This leaves the metal, now known as an ion, with a net positive charge (more protons than electrons). Metal ions—never atoms—are the only form of metal found in food.

Chelation makes it possible for metal ions to pass through cell membranes. Chelation is a process that occurs with a metal ion and another chemical—a chelator—with several special properties. Like all chemical compounds, chelators contain several different atoms joined together, but some of these atoms have electron rings that are fairly well exposed to the surroundings. These electron rings are, of course, negatively charged, which allows them to attract positively charged metal ions, as the opposite ends of magnets attract each other. Once attracted to the chelator, the smaller metal ion will then tuck itself into the part of the chelator that has the electrons exposed. Usually, two or three chelator molecules will surround the metal ion, essentially hiding the charged ion. Because these chelates have no charge, they pass unimpeded through the membrane and into the cell. In this form, the charged metal ion is figuratively "smuggled" through the protective barriers to the inside of the cell. In many instances, cells produce special "gates" or "doors" made of proteins that allow the chelator with its hidden metal ion to pass easily through the membrane walls.

Why picolinic acid? To do the job right and avoid detection, metal chelators must have atoms that attract and hide metal ions efficiently. In nature the atoms that do this best are sulfur, nitrogen and oxygen. The most common chelators contain nitrogen or oxygen or a combination of both. These atoms are the "talons" of the claw. The most efficient metal chelators are ones that have both, because most metals prefer a combination of nitrogen and oxygen. The oxygen atoms generally attract the metal ion and then direct it to and hold it in a position where the nitrogen atom can help cover up the charge on the metal ion. Metal ions are most efficiently smuggled into cells tucked inside chelators that have claws made up of four talons, usually two carbon atoms, one nitrogen and one oxygen atom. Picolinic acid is an ideal chelator because it has a nitrogen atom, an oxygen atom and two carbon atoms in close proximity, which makes it easy to hold a metal ion in a ring that has five parts: the kind most preferred.

The biological fluids that surround cells contain many kinds of charged ions and one that causes particular problems for metal ions is the positively charged hydrogen ion. Many chelators, including the overrated amino acids or links of protein, attract and hold hydrogen ions in their talons rather easily. This, of course, makes it more difficult for the metal ions to hide inside the chelator, because the holding sites become occupied by hydrogen ions. Unlike the amino acids and other potential metal chelators in the body, picolinic acid does not have holding sites or talons that strongly attract hydrogen ions. Because of this weak attraction for the charged hydrogen ions in body fluids, the nitrogen and oxygen atoms of picolinic acid do not have attached hydrogen ions and are readily available for metal chelation.

DISCOVERY OF PICOLINIC ACID IN LIVING CELLS

Scientific reports of experiments with picolinic acid first appeared over 100 years ago but, despite that early recognition, this important chemical remained virtually obscure until the latter half of this century. The early experiments with picolinic acid were done mainly by chemists who were interested in its metal-chelating properties. Chelates of picolinic acid with copper, iron, chromium and cobalt were among the first studied. These studies were later followed by others on chelation with zinc, nickel, cadmium and lead.

While these chelating experiments were being conducted, the presence of picolinic acid in human cells was apparently not known. Thus, even though chemists had been describing the excellent chelating properties of picolinic acid for years, when this chemical compound was first identified in living cells, chelation of metal ions was apparently not considered as a possible function of the compound. This lack of recognition of the importance of picolinic acid certainly cannot be attributed to stupidity on the part of the discoverers. When picolinic acid was first recognized as a cellular chemical, interest in the role of the metal ions in life processes was just beginning to emerge.

Discovery of the cellular use of picolinic acid came in the late 1970s, after scientists finally recognized the importance of metals in cellular functions and discovered that chelators control the ability of metals to enter living cells. This last and very important discovery was based on the observation of a genetic disease that prevents cells from producing a natural chelator.

Credit for the discovery of picolinic acid in the cell goes to Dr. Alan Mehler, who discovered it quite by accident.[1] He was studying enzymes that were needed for the cell to break down the essential amino acid, tryptophan. Prior to Mehler's studies, scientists had managed to trace the path of tryptophan breakdown to niacin (vitamin B3). Suspecting that not all of the tryptophan that arrived in a cell was converted to niacin and its derivatives, Mehler discovered an enzyme that directed the breakdown of tryptophan away from niacin toward the production of other cell products, one of these being picolinic acid.

This enzyme was given the simple name picolinic carboxylase, because it produced an unstable chemical that quickly rearranged itself into the stable product, picolinic acid. Despite the recognition of picolinic acid in living cells, nobody thought to measure the quantity of this chemical in the cell. All of the early studies were directed toward determining the properties of the enzyme, picolinic carboxylase, that forms picolinic acid. For that reason, in the descriptions of picolinic carboxylase, we must assume that changes in activity of this enzyme are followed directly by identical changes in the quantity of its product, picolinic acid. In other words, when the activity of the enzyme is high, the production of picolinic acid is high, and when the activity of the enzyme is low or barely detectable, the production of picolinic acid in the cell is low or absent.

When certain amino acids, particularly tryptophan, are broken down inside cells, specific side products called metabolites are made that often cannot be used by the cells. These metabolites are moved out of the cells into the blood and eventually end up in the urine. Shortly before Mehler's discovery, researchers had noticed that the urine from diabetic humans and animals contained some metabolites of tryptophan not found in the urine of normal animals and people. This encouraged Mehler and coworkers to examine the activity of picolinic carboxylase in liver tissue from diabetic rats.[2] They injected a chemical called alloxan, which destroys the cells that produce the hormone insulin and discovered that the activity of picolinic carboxylase was greatly increased in the rats which had been made diabetic. However, if rats were made diabetic with alloxan and then given regular injections of insulin, the activity of picolinic carboxylase was not increased. These experiments proved that insulin regulates the activity of picolinic carboxylase.

At that time, there was a great deal of interest in a hormone called cortisone, which is produced in a gland located on the top of the kidney called the adrenal gland. To test the effect of cortisone on picolinic carboxylase, the researchers first removed the adrenal glands from rats and, after the rats recovered from that surgery, made them diabetic with alloxan injections. When the investigators examined the activity of the enzyme, they discovered that it did not increase as it had in rats that had been made diabetic with their adrenals intact. The researchers then injected cortisone into the diabetic rats that had their adrenals removed. In these rats, the activity of picolinic carboxylase was elevated above normal, proving that the activity of the enzyme is turned on by cortisone and turned off by insulin, and therefore that cortisone increases the production of picolinic acid and insulin shuts down its production. The observations from these experiments were especially interesting to scientists because they showed that picolinic carboxylase is regulated by hormones. Enzymes that are regulated in this way often play a key role in the cell. This knowledge encouraged researchers to further examine picolinic carboxylase and also to study its product, picolinic acid.

Where picolinic acid is found in the body. Several interesting facts about picolinic carboxylase arose during the course of investigations into this enzyme.[3] The enzyme is apparently located only in the liver and kidneys, with the activity in the kidney being several times greater than that in the liver. Also, the activity of picolinic carboxylase in the kidney, unlike that of picolinic carboxylase in the liver, is not regulated by cortisone or insulin. The activity of this enzyme in other organs is either nonexistent or is so low that it is undetectable. The liver enzyme apparently varies widely in activity among species, with the highest activity being in cat liver. The significance of this observation remains to be determined.

Although the early experiments with picolinic carboxylase produced a wealth of interesting and valuable information about how the enzyme works, nothing in those experiments gave any clue to the function of or need for picolinic acid. When the early experiments on picolinic carboxylase and picolinic acid were being conducted, the *coup de grâce* for further investigations into the function of picolinic acid was probably administered when one group of investigators injected the chemical into rats and found that it was later recovered in the urine essentially intact. Since it was not degraded into another product, scientists assumed that picolinic acid was not important to cell activity, and, eventually, interest in both picolinic acid and picolinic carboxylase subsided as scientists turned their attention to more fruitful areas of research. There was no reason for investigators to suspect a chelating role for picolinic acid, since neither the role of trace metals in life functions nor the importance of metal chelators was appreciated or understood at the time.

A DETECTIVE STORY: DISCOVERY OF THE FUNCTION OF PICOLINIC ACID

Linking picolinic acid to a chelating function in the cell turned out to be like finding the villain in one of Agatha Christie's mysteries. There were clues from many sources, blind alleys and a vast array of characters, some active and some passive.

For about seven years, starting in 1971, my colleagues and I had been trying to discover how metals such as copper, chromium, iron and zinc are extracted from the diet, transported through the blood and ultimately delivered to the cells where they are stored and used. Primarily because of the ease of obtaining and working with its radioactive form, we directed much of our attention toward zinc. Our years of study proved that an organic molecule most probably secreted by the pancreas combined with zinc from the diet to transfer the metal through the membranes of the absorptive cells of the intestines. We called that molecule the zinc-binding ligand, and, for many years, the identity of the compound escaped our detection. In fact, we were very close to calling an end to our search when one of my associates brought me some research papers describing a disease called acrodermatitis enteropathica.

The plot thickens. Acrodermatitis enteropathica (AE) is a genetically transmitted disease of newborn babies that appears shortly after they have been put on a diet of infant formula. Children who have this disease develop a severe rash, have no immunity to diseases and undergo drastic behavioral changes. Untreated, the disease can lead to death. The paper of most interest to me and my associates described how a pediatrician had arrested the symptoms of AE by simply feeding his patients about five times the recommended daily allowance of zinc.[4] This suggested that the symptoms occur because the children cannot utilize the zinc normally present in the diet. We decided that there were two possible explanations for the cause of the problems: Either the children required higher levels of dietary zinc because they did not produce enough of a specific chelator needed to bind and utilize the zinc in the diet, or they did not produce enough intestinal zinc receptors. (Receptors are the parts of membranes that attract and direct specific nutrients to where they are needed for use in the body.) For several reasons—in addition to the fact that I had spent a good portion of my scientific career looking for a zinc chelator—we favored the former possibility.

After spending more time reading the research results of others than producing our own results, we agreed that at least three noteworthy points surfaced in most of the research papers related to AE. 1) The symptoms of AE occur *after* the child has been weaned from mother's milk. Also, human breast milk was used with many children to arrest the symptoms. 2) For several years a drug called hydroxyquinoline had been successfully used for the treatment of the disease. This drug was being used empirically, which means that nobody knew exactly why it worked. 3) Many of the research reports, and one in particular by an Atlanta physician, described observations which indicated that children afflicted with AE have drastically changed cellular breakdown of tryptophan.

These three pertinent observations directed the course of our thinking and research for the future. The first two observations guided us toward a zinc chelator in human breast milk. Since we knew that the zinc concentration of human milk was often less than the zinc concentration of infant formula or cow's milk, we concluded that the beneficial effects of mother's milk were not due to higher zinc intake. Because the chemical structure of the drug, hydroxyquinoline is similar to the structure of chemicals used for the analysis of zinc, we deduced that the drug could easily chelate zinc and probably substitute for a naturally produced chelator. Thus, we theorized that human milk contains a natural chelator needed to direct zinc from the intestinal contents to the cells. Because AE patients have abnormal tryptophan metabolites in their urine, we suspected that one of the compounds produced during the breakdown of tryptophan might be a zinc chelator.

Fortunately, I had in my office an old version of *Harper's Review of Physiological Chemistry*, which contained a complete diagram of the products formed during the breakdown of tryptophan. After carefully examining the structures of all the products formed when tryptophan is broken down, we were left with several prospective chelators. The prime candidates were quinolinic acid and picolinic acid, because their chemical properties were nearest to those of ideal chelators.

Success at last. Using some novel methods, we eventually isolated a zinc chelator from human milk and set out to identify the compound. Since we had two possible choices, we simply compared the properties of our isolated chelator with the properties of picolinic and quinolinic acids, and we quickly discovered that the natural product was picolinic acid. We then assayed picolinic acid in human milk, infant formula and cow's milk and discovered that only human milk contains it in measurable quantities.[5] Next, we compared the properties of the zinc chelator from the intestine with picolinic acid and realized that we had at last identified one of nature's legitimate chelators. I use the term "legitimate" because the molecule is produced in the human cell, not the test tube, for the purpose of combining with essential metals to ensure proper utilization in the body.

Shortly after we identified picolinic acid in human milk, I received a telephone call that began a collaboration which turned out to be critical for proving that picolinic acid plays an important role in the body. Dr. Inga Krieger called me about a patient she was treating who required higher than normal quantities of zinc in her daily diet. The patient, an infant girl, had developed the symptoms of AE at four months of age, after her mother had stopped breast-feeding her. Dr. Krieger started giving the infant a commercial pancreatic extract and noted that her rash and other diagnostic symptoms of AE disappeared. Later, the child was given daily supplements of oral zinc, which were effective only when the daily dose exceeded 30 mg zinc per day (a quantity twice the adult Recommended Dietary Allowance). Dr. Krieger had read one of our publications postulating the presence of a zinc chelator in the pancreas. She contacted me after she found that the quantity of zinc her patient required when she was being supplemented with the pancreatic extract, was less than 5 mg per day! We agreed to test the pancreatic extract and quickly proved that Dr. Krieger's suspicions were correct. The pancreatic extract, like human milk, was effective because it contained the zinc chelator picolinic acid.[6]

Other collaborative experiments with Dr. Krieger were equally productive. She obtained the parents' permission and started giving the same infant daily supplements of zinc picolinate that we had prepared. In this trial the girl was given only 5 mg zinc per day, which was considerably less than the 30 mg per day she had required before. The difference, of course, was that the 5 mg per day dose was administered as zinc picolinate, while the 30 mg per day dose was given as zinc sulfate. The infant remained symptom-free during the several months she was treated with zinc picolinate.

Next, Dr. Krieger enlisted the services of Dr. Ralph Cash, who was treating patients with diagnosed AE on a regular basis. The two doctors obtained the necessary permissions, discontinued treatment with oral zinc sulfate and, as soon as the rash and behavioral symptoms reappeared, started treating the patients with low doses of zinc complexed with picolinic acid. The daily zinc supplement needed by each of the children in this study was reduced considerably when the supplement was given as zinc picolinate rather than zinc sulfate.

These results were exciting and encouraging, but the most significant part of this experiment was the observation we made when we measured picolinic acid levels in the blood of these children. By using a sensitive and accurate procedure called high-performance liquid chromatography, we discovered that the plasma picolinic acid level of normal children is three to four times greater than the picolinic acid level of children with AE.[7] These analyses proved that children who inherit the faulty gene that causes AE do not produce as much picolinic acid as normal children. Since children with AE, unless given supplements of zinc picolinate, require much higher levels of daily dietary zinc than normal children to remain healthy, these experiments also proved that the body must produce sufficient quantities of picolinic acid to make efficient use of the zinc normally present in the average daily diet.

PICOLINIC ACID'S VITAL ROLE IN ZINC UTILIZATION

The experimental results obtained with AE patients were only one link in the long chain of investigations that established the role of picolinic acid in the body. The fact that this product of tryptophan breakdown is a chelator in living systems was verified by many diverse human and animal experiments. After identifying picolinic acid in human milk, we designed several experiments to determine how necessary it was in maintaining normal zinc utilization in animals. To accomplish this, we studied what happens to zinc absorption when animals are fed diets that have too little tryptophan. This was done in two different ways. We first fed rats diets that contained a suboptimal level of protein, because other investigators had observed that low-protein diets caused decreased zinc absorption. We also observed that zinc absorption was low in rats fed inadequate protein. We proved why this happens when we discovered that zinc absorption returned to normal when either tryptophan or picolinic acid was added to these diets.[8]

We then studied zinc absorption in rats fed zein, a protein from corn which has little tryptophan. Zinc absorption in the animals fed this diet was also below normal unless we added either tryptophan or picolinic acid to the diet.[9]

Several years ago, scientists studying the breakdown of tryptophan in cells discovered that vitamin B6 must be present in order for cells to properly rearrange the atoms of tryptophan into other chemicals. Thus, in order for picolinic acid to be made from tryptophan, the cells must have an adequate supply of pyridoxine (B6). After we had started our work with picolinic acid, we found a scientific report which showed that the amount of zinc in several organs was decreased if rats were fed a diet that did not have enough vitamin B6. This effect did not occur when rats were fed diets deficient in either of the vitamins thiamine (B1) or riboflavin (B2). This proved that the effect was specific for B6 and prompted us to do some similar experiments.

We were able to repeat those observations and also found that both growth and kidney zinc content could be increased markedly if picolinic acid was added to diets deficient in vitamin B6. Also, by injecting rats with radioactive zinc and waiting several days for the radioactive metal to be distributed throughout the body, we found that the body stores of zinc were managed in direct proportion to the amount of vitamin B6 in the diet. The higher the content of vitamin B6, the longer zinc remained in the body. These experiments showed that utilization of zinc by the body depends upon vitamin B6, because this vitamin helps control the conversion of tryptophan into picolinic acid.

The zinc-iron problem solved by picolinic acid. The amount of iron in a diet has a pronounced effect on how much zinc can be transferred from the intestines to the blood. In scientific terms, iron is a competitor of zinc absorption. Put simply, iron is like the schoolyard bully who sees something he wants and takes it, especially when he has a crowd of friends with him. We discovered that by adding either picolinic acid or vitamin B6 to a diet we could overcome the competition between iron and zinc. We had measured the amount of zinc absorbed into the blood in rats being fed a standard experimental diet and compared the results with the amount of zinc that was absorbed when the amount of iron in the diet was increased sevenfold.

The addition of the excess iron to the diet caused over a 30 percent decrease in the amount of zinc that was transferred from the intestines to the body. However, when either picolinic acid or an additional amount of vitamin B6 was put into the diets that contained the excess iron, the amount of zinc absorbed was actually higher than that seen when the standard diet was used.[10] This set of experiments proved that iron competes with zinc for picolinic acid in the intestines. Like the school bully and his buddies, who push the weak kid out of his seat on the bus, iron pushes zinc away from picolinic acid, and if there is not enough of the chelator in the intestine, zinc has no way of being transported to the blood.

During our experiments we also observed some dramatic effects of picolinic acid in rats that were fed supposedly adequate diets. When rats were fed a standard experimental diet with picolinic acid added, they gained more weight than rats fed the same diet without added picolinic acid. Also, the rats fed the supplemented diet absorbed more zinc and had more zinc in their kidneys than the unsupplemented rats.[11]

In another experiment, zinc was measured in baby rats whose mothers had been given either zinc picolinate or zinc acetate in their drinking water during the last five days of pregnancy and for five days while they were nursing the newborn rat pups. The amount of zinc in both the liver and kidneys was much higher in the baby rats whose mothers had been given zinc picolinate.[12]

Zinc, picolinic acid and vitamin A. Testing picolinic acid has not been confined to my laboratory or to experiments with rats. Overseas, a group of Italian investigators[13] fed one group of rats a diet that did not contain enough tryptophan and fed another group of rats a diet that had too little zinc. Both groups of rats ended up with the classical signs associated with too little zinc in the diet. These scientists proved that the effects were directly related to low tryptophan levels by feeding another group of rats a suboptimal amount of the amino acid leucine. The low-leucine diet did not cause the same effects as the low tryptophan diet. The rats fed either the low tryptophan diet or the low zinc diet had less zinc in the blood than the animals fed either a low-leucine diet or a standard diet.

Especially noteworthy was the observation of parakeratosis of the esophageal mucosa (hardening of the esophagus cells) in both the tryptophan-deficient rats and the zinc-deficient rats. We now know that mucus-secreting cells like those in the esophagus require vitamin A for proper function. When vitamin A is not delivered to these cells, they produce a protein called keratin, which makes the cells harder and less pliable. Vitamin A is stored in the liver and requires a specific protein in order to be transported to the cells where it is needed. Zinc is absolutely necessary for the production of this vitamin A transport protein. These scientists prevented the rats from transferring adequate amounts of zinc into the body by simply stopping the production of picolinic acid. This eventually led to the same effects as a low-zinc diet, the accumulation of keratin in certain cells resulting from insufficient vitamin A.

Picolinic acid and pellagra. Drs. Inga Krieger and Marion Statter also showed that lack of tryptophan in the diet affects zinc levels in the body.[14] They studied rats fed diets deficient in tryptophan and noted that blood and bone zinc were decreased. When picolinic acid was added to the diet, plasma and bone zinc levels were restored to normal.

These authors discussed the fact that their study provides evidence that the nutritional deficiency disease pellagra may be caused by a lack of picolinic acid production in the body. Pellagra is a nutritional disease found in people whose food does not contain enough tryptophan.

Pellagrans have poorly developed skin and hair and also have intestinal problems similar to those of people who do not take enough zinc from their diet. Pellagra has been traditionally linked to a deficiency in niacin (B3), even though pellagra often occurs in people who have adequate levels of niacin in their diets. The experiments of Krieger and Statter explain this paradox and show that pellagra is most probably caused by the low production of picolinic acid because of insufficient tryptophan. The decreased amount of picolinic acid would lessen the amount of zinc absorbed from the diet and cause the skin, hair and intestinal problems.

Other studies on picolinic acid and zinc. In what are probably the most recent studies with the enzyme picolinic carboxylase, Drs. Statter and Krieger discovered that the action of the enzyme in the liver increases during pregnancy, drops off just before giving birth and then increases markedly while the mother is nursing.[15] This experiment shows that more picolinic acid is made during pregnancy, allowing essential metals to be transported to the fetus developing in the womb. During the nursing period, more picolinic acid is produced in the mother so that adequate amounts of the metal chelator are present in the milk to deliver metal ions to the body of the nursing newborn.

In England, Seal and Heaton conducted extensive studies with picolinic acid.[16] These investigators studied zinc transfer through intestinal cells of rats. They assayed zinc sulfate, zinc chloride, zinc acetate, zinc citrate, zinc aspartate (an amino acid chelate), zinc histidinate (another amino acid chelate) and zinc picolinate. The uptake of zinc picolinate by the intestinal cells was several times greater than the uptake of the other forms of zinc.

They also found that an altered form of picolinic acid, one that can be produced in the test tube but not in the body, actually decreased the uptake of zinc. This observation gives us some evidence that cells may have special "gates" for transferring the naturally occurring forms of metal picolinates through the cell membranes. Seal and Heaton also proved that picolinic acid added to the diet of rats increases the absorption as well as the excretion of zinc. This observation prompted them to warn against the indiscriminate use of picolinic acid to prevent or cure metal deficiencies. This is discussed in more detail on pages 22–23.

Observations in humans, other than those obtained in children afflicted with acrodermatitis enteropathica, have provided more evidence to prove the importance of the metal chelating function of naturally produced picolinic acid. Dr. Phyllis Johnson proved that zinc absorption is decreased in humans fed a diet low, but not actually deficient, in tryptophan.[17] While consuming this diet, individuals absorbed only 56 percent of the zinc present. This contrasts strongly with the 92 percent absorption of dietary zinc by individuals consuming a balanced diet containing adequate tryptophan.

These observations raise some interesting points for future consideration by the committees who establish the Recommended Dietary Allowance (RDA) for human beings. Although the test diet contained what the study's results indicate to be a low quantity of tryptophan (235 mg per day by calculation), it was not, going by the current RDA of 210 mg, actually deficient in tryptophan. Yet when individuals were fed a similar diet with substantial additional quantities of tryptophan, zinc absorption increased greatly. Since picolinic acid in the body is produced only from tryptophan, this study provides yet another link between this amino acid and metal utilization. In view of these observations, is it possible that the current RDA for tryptophan is too low?

In a carefully controlled experiment conducted at the Veterans Administration Medical Center in Minneapolis, Maria Boosalis and Dr. Craig McClain proved that a normally functioning pancreas is necessary for proper zinc absorption in humans.[18] Health employees and patients with various diseases of the liver, intestines and other organs served as controls. These people and five patients with diseases of the pancreas were all given an oral dose of zinc sulfate. Blood was drawn at intervals to measure how fast zinc was being transported into the body. Two days later, the same people were given an oral dose of zinc picolinate and zinc transfer into the blood was again measured. When compared with healthy individuals, patients with pancreatic diseases showed very low zinc absorption from zinc sulfate. However, zinc absorption from zinc picolinate was normal in these patients. Thus, healthy individuals store picolinic acid in the pancreas, and it can then be secreted into the intestines to chelate metal ions from the diet for transfer into the blood. People with a diseased pancreas cannot store or secrete picolinic acid during ingestion of food, so the transfer of zinc and probably other metals into the body is decreased.

Zinc picolinate assimilates best—no contest. Dr. Stephen Barrie and his associates conducted an in-depth study which proved that zinc picolinate is the most effective form of zinç supplementation.[19] Healthy students took oral supplements of zinc picolinate, zinc citrate, zinc gluconate and a placebo. Every student was first given one of the supplement forms for a period of four weeks. After a two-week waiting period with no supplements, the students were then given another form of supplement for four weeks, followed by another two-week waiting period. This was continued until everyone had used each of the four different types of supplements for four weeks.

This is the most meaningful experimental design because each of the students served as his own control.

Zinc was measured in hair, urine and red blood cells and serum at the beginning and again at the end of each supplement period. During supplementation with zinc picolinate, zinc increased in hair, urine and red blood cells. No meaningful increases were observed in any of these during supplementation with zinc citrate, zinc gluconate or the placebo.

Dr. Barrie's study is particularly noteworthy because the supplements were taken three times per day, between meals, which means that competing metals such as iron, copper, chromium and manganese were present in the intestinal contents. The zinc ions released from citrate and gluconate would be forced to compete with these other metals for the picolinic acid secreted from the pancreas, and the quantity of zinc transferred into the blood would be decreased. By contrast, when the supplement contained zinc picolinate, the metal arrived at the absorption sites of the intestine in a form ready to be transferred into the body. Thus, as this study illustrates, the most efficient and, therefore, beneficial form of supplementation occurs when metals are combined with a naturally produced chelator which is quickly recognized by body cells.

CHROMIUM AND OTHER METAL PICOLINATES

The scientific experiments described thus far show that picolinic acid is a very effective chelator. These discussions may tend to give the impression that it is only effective with zinc. But picolinic acid also combines easily with cobalt, copper, chromium, iron, manganese and nickel. I have observed beneficial effects from supplementation with iron picolinate, copper picolinate, manganese picolinate and chromium picolinate. Many of the observations with other metal picolinates were taken from piecemeal experiments with rats and, although significant, do not have the health implications of our tests in humans with chromium picolinate.

Several years ago, while my associates and I were studying metal absorption, we gave different radioactive metals orally to rats that had been fed a diet low in zinc; the idea was to measure how much of each metal was absorbed if the rat's body was depleted of zinc. We noted that the zinc-deficient rats absorbed far more radioactive chromium than rats fed an adequate amount of zinc.

When we mixed zinc with radioactive chromium before giving it to the rats, the absorption of chromium was greatly decreased. And when we mixed chromium with radioactive zinc before giving it to the rats, absorption of the zinc was decreased.[20] To my knowledge, this was the first and perhaps the last experiment done to test an interaction between zinc and chromium, but the results proved that these two minerals antagonize each other in the intestine. At that time, the real meaning of those observations was not apparent but, after we identified picolinic acid in cellular fluid, one of the first metals I studied—other than zinc—was chromium.

There were two basic reasons for this interest: one, of course, was the interaction we had observed years before, and the other was a set of experimental results published by scientists with the USDA in Beltsville, Maryland. These investigators claimed that chromium in cells was combined with nicotinic acid, which is another name for vitamin B3 or niacin.[21] Nicotinic acid is what chemists call an isomer of picolinic acid. That means that nicotinic acid is similar, but not identical, to picolinic acid. Even though nicotinic acid is similar to picolinic acid, it is inferior as a metal chelator, so I questioned the validity of those observations and began studying combinations of chromium and picolinic acid.

We first made chromium picolinate with radioactive chromium. Chromium picolinate consists of one chromium atom surrounded by three molecules of picolinic acid. We tested this compound in rats and observed that chromium picolinate is absorbed far better than chromium chloride. We then began human experiments in the fall of 1988 in collaboration with Dr. Ray Press at Mercy Hospital in San Diego, California.

Prior to these studies, research results from several investigators had suggested that chromium plays a role in maintaining normal fat and carbohydrate levels in body tissues and fluid.[22] This hypothesis had previously been difficult to confirm because chromium, unless combined with the proper chelator, is absorbed poorly by humans and animals. The suggested daily intake for chromium is 50 to 200 micrograms, and estimates have been made that 90 percent of Americans do not consume adequate amounts of this mineral. Several studies have shown that efficient absorption of chromium occurs only when the metal is combined with a specific chemical made in kidney and in certain yeasts. Since these food items clearly are not staples of modern diets, many investigators have attempted to isolate and identify a chemical transporter that will improve the utilization of chromium.

We know that picolinic acid is an effective metal chelator, made from tryptophan in mammalian kidney cells. One of my students proved that picolinic acid is also made in brewer's yeast. Thus, Dr. Press and I designed a series of experiments to test the effectiveness of chromium picolinate in humans.

Chromium picolinate and cholesterol. In the 1988 Mercy Hospital study, 28 volunteers were given either chromium picolinate—which contained 200 mcg of chromium—or a placebo daily for 42 days, followed by a 14-day period with no treatment. Each of the volunteers then served as his or her own control by taking the supplement not used in the first trial period. Blood was drawn at the beginning, at three weeks and again at the end of each 42-day treatment period. A complete analysis was obtained on the blood drawn at the beginning and the end, so those were the values used to determine the results of the study.

Although no meaningful changes were observed while the people were given the placebo, several significant results were obtained during supplementation with chromium picolinate. When the volunteers were supplemented with chromium picolinate, total cholesterol and low-density lipoprotein cholesterol (the "bad" cholesterol) decreased significantly. Total cholesterol for the experimental groups decreased 7 percent from an average of 276 milligrams per deciliter of blood to 256 mg/dl, while LDL-cholesterol decreased 10.5 percent from 200 mg/dl to 178 mg/dl during treatment with chromium picolinate. Of the final 28 volunteers, 22 had lower total cholesterol, two were unchanged and the remaining four had cholesterol concentrations elevated less than 5 mg/dl. Twenty individuals had decreased concentrations of LDL-cholesterol, three were unchanged and the others had slightly elevated concentrations. The concentration of serum high-density lipoprotein cholesterol (the "good" kind) increased slightly in the period during which the subjects were ingesting chromium picolinate. These observations were encouraging because elevated blood cholesterol (hypercholesterolemia) has been linked to death from heart disease.

Particularly relevant was the decrease in LDL-cholesterol, the medical label given the form of cholesterol that enters the blood from the liver as determined by the diet. Normally, the body uses a portion of dietary cholesterol for body needs. In fact, the body uses and replenishes about 2,000 mg of cholesterol daily. The remainder of the cholesterol from the diet is broken down or stored in the cells. When storage and breakdown cannot keep pace with what the body absorbs from the diet or produces (if the person does not take in 2,000 mg or so from the diet, the body has to manufacture the difference), the cholesterol floats around in the blood in the form of LDL-cholesterol, the "bad" kind, which gets deposited in the blood vessels.

When cholesterol first enters the body from the diet, it is delivered to the liver. There it is broken down, utilized for body functions or stored. When the storage capacity of the liver is exceeded, the cholesterol is attached to a protein called apolipoprotein B (apo B), which carries the cholesterol to other cells of the body. The more cholesterol that must be transported, the greater the production of apo B. During treatment with chromium picolinate, apo B, the LDL fraction, decreased very significantly. This shows that chromium picolinate supplements caused a great enough decrease in liver cholesterol to signal the body to cut back on production of the transport protein. Chromium picolinate caused either an increased breakdown of cholesterol in the liver, an accelerated uptake of cholesterol by cells outside the liver, a decreased absorption of dietary cholesterol, or perhaps a combination of all these.

Cholesterol, in spite of what one might read in the press, is a very important chemical in the body. Every cell uses some cholesterol, but some cells use more than others. The liver uses large amounts of cholesterol to make special chemicals used for digestion of food. To transport cholesterol from storage cells in the body to the cells where it is needed—especially in the liver—the body produces a protein called apolipoprotein A1. The appearance of this protein in the blood is a signal that the body is using cholesterol that has been stored or produced in cells outside the liver. This is an indication that the body is keeping ahead of or at least in step with the dietary intake and liver production of cholesterol. The cholesterol attached to this protein is HDL-cholesterol, the beneficial kind. Some experts believe that the HDL fraction actually helps remove cholesterol that may have been deposited in blood vessels. In our study, apolipoprotein A1 increased significantly during treatment with chromium picolinate.

Chromium picolinate and diabetes. In a second study at Mercy Hospital, identical in design to the one discussed on pages 18-19, 11 diabetic volunteers were given either chromium picolinate or a placebo. These patients had diabetes mellitus, which is the most common form of the disease and is caused by either the body's inability to produce the hormone insulin or to utilize the insulin that is produced. The primary function of insulin is to cause glucose (blood sugar) to be taken up by certain cells. When insulin is not present or cannot be used properly, glucose accumulates in the blood until it reaches high levels (hyperglycemia). One of the side effects of this accumulation is frequent urination; the kidneys excrete the excess glucose, which takes water with it.

A chemical reaction that occurs between glucose and proteins in the body is being studied extensively today. Normally, very little glucose combines with proteins, but when the quantity of glucose is very high in the blood, as in diabetes mellitus, protein does combine with glucose. One of the proteins that reacts with glucose is the oxygen-carrying protein hemoglobin. When glucose reacts with it, the protein acquires different chemical properties than normal hemoglobin and it can be easily detected in the blood. This new protein is called hemoglobin A_1C or glycosylated hemoglobin (hemoglobin with glucose attached), and it is used to detect changes in insulin action in the body. In our study, both glycosylated hemoglobin and fasting blood glucose decreased significantly during supplementation with chromium picolinate. This observation proves that the chromium from chromium picolinate or perhaps the whole compound somehow improved the action of insulin in the patients we studied.

In both human studies, potentially harmful blood chemicals (elevated levels of cholesterol and glucose) were decreased after only six weeks with daily supplements of the naturally occurring nutrient chromium picolinate. Chromium picolinate is inexpensive, safe and nontoxic. Combined with a prudent regulation of diet, chromium picolinate could be used as an adjunct to the treatment and prevention of heart disease and diabetes.

Chromium picolinate and muscle development—an alternative to steroids. Greatly encouraged by the results of the first two human studies, Dr. Muriel Gilman, who is an exercise physiologist at Bemidji State University, Minnesota, and I conducted an experiment to study the effect of chromium picolinate on muscle development, which was completed in February 1989. Students recruited from weight-training classes offered at the university were given, at random, either a placebo or chromium picolinate, and instructed to consume one capsule per day for 40 days. The identity of the capsules was known only to an individual not participating in the trial. The placebo capsules contained only calcium phosphate, while the chromium capsules contained calcium phosphate and chromium picolinate (200 micrograms of chromium). At the start and end of the trial, height and weight, as well as biceps and calf circumferences, were measured. Also, the thickness of the skin (skinfold) was measured on various parts of the body to calculate the amount of muscle in the body, which physiologists call lean body mass. During the course of the trial, the students maintained their normal dietary and activity habits while participating in a prescribed weight-lifting program three hours a week.

The circumference of both the biceps and calf increased more in the students taking chromium picolinate than in those who took the placebo. In the chromium picolinate group, biceps circumference increased by an average of 1.4 cm (0.55 inch), while the placebo group biceps increase was 1.2 cm (0.47 inch). The calf circumference of the students who took chromium picolinate increased an average of 1.15 cm (0.45 inch), but the increase was only 0.82 cm (0.32 inch) in the placebo group. The body weight of the students given chromium picolinate increased about 4¾ pounds, while that of the students given the placebo increased about 2½ pounds. The calculated increase in lean body mass of the students taking chromium picolinate was about 3½ pounds, but the increase with the placebo group was less than 2 ounces. This shows that nearly three-fourths of the weight gain in the students given chromium picolinate was lean muscle. Although this was a preliminary study, the observations raise a strong possibility that chromium picolinate can be used as a safe alternative to anabolic steroids. (Note: As this booklet was going to press, we completed a second study involving over 30 athletes and found nearly identical results.)

Chromium picolinate enhances the function of insulin. The experimental results seen with chromium picolinate could lead the uninitiated to think that this chemical is some kind of "snake oil" elixir, but all of the results have a strong scientific basis that can be linked to one important chemical in the body—insulin. When a person eats a meal, carbohydrates (mainly glucose), lipids (cholesterol and other forms of fat) and amino acids from protein enter the blood. Insulin is secreted from the pancreas cells to act as a chemical policeman to direct these food products to the cells where they can either be used immediately or stored for later use. Insulin can apparently do this job to some extent by itself, but many experiments show that it can do the job far more efficiently when a chromium compound acting as a co-hormone is present in adequate quantities in the body. All of the experiments we have conducted lead me to believe that this long-sought co-hormone is indeed chromium picolinate.

CAUTION

Because of their potency, a word of caution is in order regarding the use of metal picolinates. The caution is directed to both professionals and the general public, because the use of mineral picolinates will necessitate some careful considerations of metal requirements. One must remember that the recommended daily intake (RDA) for each of the minerals is much higher than the quantity actually used in the body. This is because the minerals that enter the intestine from the diet must either already be attached to a suitable chelator or compete with other metals for the chelators present. Often, because of their positive charge, minerals combine with fiber in the diet, and this makes them unavailable for use by the body. The mineral RDA is therefore elevated to help people realize how much must be ingested to ensure that enough reaches the blood and cells to prevent deficiencies. Because minerals complexed with picolinic acid are readily absorbed and utilized by the body, less of the actual mineral is needed to satisfy cellular needs. The body requirements of metals combined with picolinic acid *is probably about one-third the requirement of an unchelated form.*

A good rule of thumb for use of the mineral picolinates would be to divide by three the RDA for the mineral or minerals in question and use only that quantity as a daily supplement. For example, the RDA for zinc is 15 mg per day, but a supplement that contained only 5 mg zinc *as zinc picolinate* would be adequate.

I have talked with several physicians who were supplementing elderly people with 15 mg zinc per day as zinc picolinate and noted that the people became anemic after a few months. This was caused by a buildup of zinc inside the cells, which eventually interfered with the utilization of iron. The problem was quickly corrected by reducing the dosage to one 15 mg supplement every other day, cutting the amount received in half. (My opinion is that 15 mg of zinc picolinate every third day would have been as effective.) Responsible companies—those truly interested in the health and welfare of the consumer—will market metal picolinates only in amounts that are safe.

As far as I know, uncomplexed or free picolinic acid is not available for human consumption and probably never will be. *Indiscriminate and uncontrolled use of picolinic acid as a food supplement could easily cause more problems than it would ever correct.* Long-term ingestion of picolinic acid could initially elevate the absorption of minerals but, eventually, the body would become saturated with excess picolinic acid, which might prevent minerals from being incorporated into cellular systems where they are required.

Also, because picolinic acid combines with several different metals, use of the free form *could lead to elevated levels of some very undesirable minerals such as cadmium and lead in the body.* For that matter, both iron and copper are extremely toxic in excessive quantities, and conditions leading to increased uptake by the blood should be avoided. One study with mice showed that high levels of picolinic acid cause destruction of kidney cells. FOR SAFETY, INGESTION OF UNCOMPLEXED PICOLINIC ACID SHOULD BE AVOIDED.

> A patent for dietary supplementation of essential metal picolinates was issued to Dr. Gary Evans in 1982 and assigned to the United States Department of Agriculture. Research and product development rights have been licensed to Nutrition 21 of San Diego, California.

CONCLUSION

Metal ions are absolutely essential for maximum performance of the body's cells. These metal ions must be extracted from the diet, moved into the blood and delivered to the cells before they can be utilized. Research shows that the body produces special chemicals called chelators to deliver the mineral ions to the cells. The body makes picolinic acid to transport the essential metals zinc, chromium, iron and manganese.

Suboptimal quantities of mineral ions in the diet cause deficiencies, but, just as often, mineral deficiencies are caused by the body's inability to transport what is in the diet to the cells where the metals are needed. Because the body depends on picolinic acid for proper absorption and utilization of some essential minerals, conditions that slow the production of this chelator also prevent optimal performance of the body cells. In apparently healthy people, this can be caused by a limited amount of tryptophan or vitamin B6, both of which are sometimes low in human diets.

Synthetic mineral picolinates are extremely useful for correcting and preventing deficiencies of specific essential minerals. Because they are identical to those formed inside the body, synthetic metal picolinates are quickly recognized and utilized by the cells.

REFERENCES

1. A.H. Mehler. Formation of picolinic and quinolinic acids following enzymatic oxidation of 3-hydroxyanthranilic acid. *Journal of Biological Chemistry* 218:241–254, 1956.
2. A.H. Mehler, E.G. McDaniel, and J.M. Hundley. Changes in the enzymatic composition of liver. II. Influence of hormones on picolinic carboxylase and tryptophan peroxidase. *Journal of Biological Chemistry* 232:331–335, 1958.
3. G.W. Evans. The role of picolinic acid in metal metabolism. *Life Chemistry Reports* 1:57–67, 1982.

4. E.J. Moynahan. Acrodermatitis enteropathica: a lethal inherited human zinc deficiency disorder. *Lancet*, 2:399–400, 1974.
5. G.W. Evans and P.E. Johnson. Characterization and quantitation of a zinc-binding ligand in human milk. *Pediatric Research* 14: 876–880, 1980.
6. I. Krieger and G.W. Evans. A variant of acrodermatitis enteropathica without hypozincemia. Therapeutic effect of a pancreatic enzyme preparation due to a zinc binding ligand. *Journal of Pediatrics* 96: 32–35, 1980.
7. I. Krieger, R. Cash, and G.W. Evans. Picolinic acid in acrodermatitis enteropathica: evidence for a disorder of tryptophan metabolism. *Journal of Pediatric Gastroenterology and Nutrition* 3:62–68, 1984.
8. G.W. Evans and E.C. Johnson. Zinc absorption in rats fed a low protein diet and a low protein diet supplemented with tryptophan or picolinic acid. *Journal of Nutrition* 110:1076–1080, 1980.
9. G.W. Evans. Normal and abnormal zinc absorption in man and animals: the tryptophan connection. *Nutrition Reviews* 38:137–141, 1980.
10. G.W. Evans and E.C. Johnson. Effect of iron, vitamin B-6 and picolinic acid on zinc absorption in the rat. *Journal of Nutrition* 111: 68–75, 1981.
11. G.W. Evans and E.C. Johnson. Growth stimulating effect of picolinic acid added to rat diets. *Proceedings of the Society for Experimental Biology and Medicine* 165:457–461, 1980.
12. G.W. Evans and E.C. Johnson. Zinc concentrations of liver and kidneys from rat pups nursing dams fed supplemental zinc dipicolinate or zinc acetate. *Journal of Nutrition* 110:2121–2124, 1980.
13. S. Seri, E. Aquilio, A. Continenza, and G. Ricciardi. Effects of dietary tryptophan bioavailability on zinc absorption in rats. *IRCS Medical Science* 12:452–453, 1984.
14. I. Krieger and M. Statter. Tryptophan deficiency and picolinic acid: effect on zinc metabolism and clinical manifestations of pellagra. *American Journal of Clinical Nutrition* 46:511–517, 1987.
15. M. Statter and I. Krieger. Picolinic carboxylase activity in rat liver and kidney. I. Influence of growth, sex, gestation, lactation, and nutritional imbalance. *Journal of Pediatric Gastroenterology and Nutrition* 2:166–170, 1983.
16. C.J. Seal and F.W. Heaton. Chemical factors affecting the intestinal absorption of zinc in vitro and in vivo. *British Journal of Nutrition* 50:317–324, 1983.
17. P.E. Johnson, G.W. Evans, and J.R. Hunt. The effect of picolinic acid supplementation on zinc absorption by men fed a low tryptophan diet. *Nutrition Research* 8:119–127, 1988.
18. M.G. Boosalis, G.W. Evans and C.J. McClain. Impaired handling of orally administered zinc in pancreatic insufficiency. *American Journal of Clinical Nutrition* 37:268–271, 1983.

19. S.A. Barrie, J.V. Wright, J.E. Pizzorno, E. Kutter, and P.C. Barron. Comparative absorption of zinc picolinate, zinc citrate and zinc gluconate in humans. *Agents and Actions* 5:1–6, 1986.
20. C.J. Hahn and G.W. Evans. Absorption of trace metals in the zinc-deficient rat. *American Journal of Physiology* 228:1020–1023, 1975.
21. E.W. Toepfer, W. Mertz, M.M. Polansky, E.E. Roginski, and W.R. Wolf. Synthetic organic chromium complexes and glucose tolerance. *Journal of Agriculture and Food Science* 25:162–165, 1977.
22. F.X. Pi-Sunyer and E.G. Offenbacher. Chromium. *Nutrition Reviews' Present Knowledge in Nutrition* 5:571–586, 1984.